GITALMAN SYNDROME NUTRITION

Comprehensive Guide on Nutritional Management and Lifestyle Strategies, Unraveling the Complexities, from Diagnosis to Delicious Low-Sodium Recipes and Beyond

Dr. Holmgren Alfred

Copyright © Holmgren Alfred 2024.

All rights reserved.

This publication may not be reproduced, distributed, or transmitted in any form or by any means, including photocopying, recording, or other electronic or mechanical methods, without the publisher's written permission, except for brief quotations in critical reviews and other copyright-permitted non-commercial uses. Contact publisher Information for permissions.

This book is fictitious. Authors create names, people, places, and events.

Any resemblance to real events, places, or people—living or dead—is coincidental.

before making any decisions or taking any actions based on the information provided in this book. The author and publisher of this book are not liable for any consequences resulting from the use of the information contained herein.

All efforts have been made to ensure the accuracy and reliability of the information presented in this book; however, the author and publisher do not warrant the completeness, timeliness, or accuracy of the information, and thus disclaim any liability arising from reliance on the information provided in this book.

Gitelman Syndrome Nutrition: With Expert Guidance" is a must-have resource for anyone dealing with Gitelman Syndrome, a rare genetic disorder that affects electrolyte balance in the body. This book is a beacon of knowledge and empowerment for patients, caregivers, and healthcare professionals alike, explaining the complexities of the condition and providing practical nutritional management strategies.

The book's central focus is a thorough examination of Gitelman Syndrome, including its causes, symptoms, diagnosis, and treatment choices. Readers acquire a thorough awareness of the condition's complexities, giving them the knowledge, they need to properly handle its hurdles.

The book's focus on nutritional considerations in Gitelman Syndrome management is central to its mission. By highlighting essential nutrients such as sodium, potassium, magnesium, and calcium, it elucidates their critical roles in maintaining electrolyte balance and outlines recommended intake levels and dietary sources. Armed with this information, readers can make informed choices to optimize their nutritional status and improve their overall well-being.

The book not only provides theoretical knowledge but also practical advice for implementing dietary strategies tailored specifically for Gitelman Syndrome. From balancing electrolytes to managing fluid intake and customizing meal plans, readers receive actionable advice supported by evidence-based recommendations. Additionally, supplementation considerations and practical tips for grocery shopping and cooking empower readers to take control of their nutrition with confidence.

The book empowers readers to cultivate a lifestyle conducive to optimal health and well-being by fostering a sense of empowerment and agency. By embracing a holistic approach to wellness, the book broadens its scope to include lifestyle factors critical for effectively managing Gitelman Syndrome. Readers learn the significance of exercise, stress management techniques, and the importance of building a strong support network.

Furthermore, the book emphasizes the importance of regular monitoring and adjustment in Gitelman Syndrome management. By emphasizing the need for ongoing follow-ups with healthcare providers and providing insights into recognizing signs of electrolyte imbalance, the book gives readers the tools they need to proactively manage their condition and mitigate potential risks.

In addition to being a practical guide, "Gitelman Syndrome Nutrition: With Expert Guidance" is a gateway to a wealth of additional resources and further reading.

By curating a list of recommended books, websites, and support groups, the book fosters a sense of community and collaboration, empowering readers to embark on their journey to optimal health armed with knowledge, support, and expertise.

CHAPTER 1
UNDERSTANDING GITELMAN SYNDROME.

Introduction to Gitelman Syndrome:

Gitelman syndrome, a rare genetic disorder characterized by electrolyte imbalances, particularly low levels of potassium and magnesium in the blood, as well as low levels of calcium and chloride, was first described by Dr. Hillel Gitelman in 1966, hence the name. It is considered an inherited renal tubular disorder, primarily affecting the kidneys' ability to reabsorb certain electrolytes, resulting in their excessive loss through urine.

Causes and symptoms:

The primary cause of Gitelman syndrome is mutations in the SLC12A3 gene, which encodes the thiazide-sensitive sodium-chloride cotransporter (NCC) in the distal convoluted tubules of the kidneys.

These mutations disrupt the function of NCC, impairing the kidneys' ability to reabsorb sodium, chloride, potassium, and magnesium from the urine, leading to their excessive excretion. Gitelman syndrome is inherited in an autosomal recessive pattern, meaning that affected individuals inherit two copies of the mutated gene, one from each parent. However, not all individuals with mutations in the SLC12A3 gene develop symptoms of Gitelman syndrome, suggesting that other genetic or environmental factors may influence the condition's expression. The hallmark symptoms of Gitelman syndrome include muscle weakness and cramps, fatigue, salt cravings, tetany (muscle spasms and twitching), dizziness, and occasionally, episodes of paralysis or arrhythmias due to severe electrolyte imbalances.

Additionally, some individuals may experience polyuria (excessive urination) and polydipsia (excessive thirst) as a compensatory mechanism to maintain electrolyte balance.

Diagnosis and treatment options:

Diagnosing Gitelman syndrome can be challenging due to its nonspecific symptoms and overlap with other electrolyte disorders such as Bartter syndrome and Liddle syndrome. However, a combination of clinical evaluation, laboratory tests, and genetic testing can help confirm the diagnosis. Laboratory findings typically reveal hypokalemia (low potassium levels), hypomagnesemia (low magnesium levels), metabolic alkalosis (elevated blood pH), and increased urinary excretion of potassium and magnesium.

Genetic testing can identify mutations in the SLC12A3 gene, further confirming the diagnosis. Once diagnosed, the main goal of treatment for Gitelman syndrome is to correct electrolyte imbalances, prevent symptoms, and minimize long-term complications.

This typically involves oral supplementation with potassium and magnesium salts to maintain normal serum levels, as well as dietary modifications to increase intake of these electrolytes.

In some cases, medications such as potassium-sparing diuretics or nonsteroidal anti-inflammatory drugs (NSAIDs) may be prescribed to help manage symptoms and reduce urinary electrolyte losses.

Nutritional Considerations for Gitelman Syndrome Management:

Nutrition plays a crucial role in managing Gitelman syndrome by optimizing electrolyte balance and supporting overall health and well-being.

Since individuals with Gitelman syndrome have increased urinary losses of potassium and magnesium, maintaining adequate intake of these electrolytes is essential to prevent deficiencies and associated symptoms.

Foods rich in potassium include bananas, oranges, potatoes, tomatoes, spinach, and avocados, while magnesium-rich foods include nuts, seeds, whole grains, leafy greens, and legumes.

However, it's important to note that potassium and magnesium supplements should be used cautiously and under medical supervision, as excessive intake can lead to hyperkalemia (high potassium levels) or hypermagnesemia (high magnesium levels), which can be dangerous. In addition to electrolyte balance, managing sodium intake is also important in Gitelman syndrome, as excessive sodium consumption can exacerbate electrolyte imbalances and increase the risk of hypertension and cardiovascular complications.

Therefore, individuals with Gitelman syndrome are typically advised to follow a low-sodium diet, which involves minimizing processed and packaged foods, avoiding added salt, and choosing fresh, whole foods whenever possible.

Furthermore, adequate hydration is essential to support kidney function and prevent dehydration, particularly during episodes of increased fluid loss through sweating, vomiting, or diarrhea. Overall, a balanced and varied diet, rich in fruits, vegetables, whole grains, and lean proteins, can help optimize nutritional status and improve outcomes for individuals with Gitelman syndrome.

CHAPTER 2
ESSENTIAL NUTRIENTS FOR GITELMAN SYNDROME

In Gitelman Syndrome (GS), a rare genetic disorder characterized by renal tubular defects affecting electrolyte handling, particularly sodium, potassium, magnesium, and calcium, sodium is vital for maintaining fluid balance, nerve function, and muscle contraction, all of which are essential physiological processes. In GS patients, renal sodium wasting causes hyponatremia, or low blood sodium levels, which contributes to symptoms.

Potassium, another essential nutrient, is intricately involved in cellular function, particularly in maintaining membrane potential and regulating muscle contraction. In Gitelman Syndrome, renal potassium wasting occurs alongside sodium wasting, leading to hypokalemia or low potassium levels in the blood. Hypokalemia can manifest as symptoms such as weakness, muscle cramps, and cardiac arrhythmias, so GS patients must ensure an adequate intake of

Magnesium deficiency is frequently observed in individuals with Gitelman Syndrome due to renal magnesium wasting. Magnesium plays a vital role in numerous physiological processes, including energy metabolism, muscle and nerve function, and bone health. Magnesium deficiency can exacerbate symptoms such as muscle weakness, tremors, and cardiac arrhythmias, so it is essential to monitor magnesium levels and ensure adequate intake through dietary sources.

Although calcium is less frequently discussed in the context of Gitelman Syndrome, it is still important for bone health and muscle function. Renal calcium wasting can occur in GS patients, potentially leading to hypocalcemia or low blood calcium levels. While the impact of calcium imbalance in GS is less pronounced than that of sodium, potassium, or magnesium, maintaining adequate calcium intake remains essential for overall health.

In conclusion, understanding the role of essential nutrients such as sodium, potassium, magnesium, and calcium is crucial in effectively managing Gitelman Syndrome. While renal tubular defects lead to electrolyte imbalances in GS patients, optimizing dietary intake and, if necessary, supplementation can help alleviate symptoms and improve overall quality of life. Close monitoring and individualized approaches are paramount to ensure adequate nutrient levels while minimizing.

CHAPTER 3
DIETARY STRATEGIES FOR GITELMAN SYNDROME MANAGEMENT

Dietary management is critical for individuals with Gitelman syndrome, a rare genetic disorder that affects electrolyte balance in the body. One fundamental aspect of dietary strategies for managing Gitelman syndrome is balancing electrolytes, particularly the sodium-potassium ratio. Electrolytes are essential minerals that play vital roles in various physiological processes, including muscle contraction, nerve conduction, and fluid balance.

Individuals with Gitelman syndrome may be prone to excessive fluid loss through increased urine output, known as polyuria, so it is essential to ensure adequate fluid intake to prevent dehydration and electrolyte imbalances. Patients are encouraged to drink water.

Individualized meal planning is essential for effectively managing Gitelman syndrome, as dietary needs may vary among patients. Customizing diets to meet the specific requirements of each individual can help optimize electrolyte balance and overall health. Working closely with a registered dietitian who is knowledgeable about Gitelman syndrome can provide personalized guidance and support in meal planning. Dietitians can help patients identify foods rich in potassium,

Supplementation considerations are also important in Gitelman syndrome management, particularly regarding vitamin and mineral supplements. Due to the increased risk of electrolyte deficiencies, patients may require supplementation to maintain optimal levels of potassium, magnesium, and other essential nutrients. However, it is essential to be cautious with supplementation because certain vitamins and minerals may interact with medications commonly used to manage Gitelman syndrome.

dietary strategies play a crucial role in managing Gitelman syndrome, a complex disorder characterized by electrolyte imbalances. Balancing electrolytes, managing fluid intake, individualizing meal plans, and considering supplementation are all essential aspects of dietary management for Gitelman syndrome.

Patients can optimize their diets to support overall health by collaborating with healthcare professionals, particularly registered dietitians.

CHAPTER 4
PRACTICAL TIPS AND RECIPES

Gitelman Syndrome, a rare genetic disorder affecting the kidneys, presents unique challenges in managing one's diet and lifestyle due to its impact on electrolyte balance, particularly sodium, potassium, magnesium, and calcium. To address these challenges, practical tips and recipes play a crucial role in assisting individuals with Gitelman Syndrome to navigate their nutritional needs effectively. This section delves into various aspects of practical tips and recipes tailored

Grocery Shopping with Gitelman Syndrome:

Foods labeled as "low-sodium" or "so" require careful inspection to accurately identify sodium content, as excessive sodium intake worsens symptoms like muscle weakness, fatigue, and irregular heartbeat in Gitelman Syndrome patients.

Cooking methods for electrolyte retention:

Certain cooking techniques, such as boiling, steaming, and simmering, can help preserve electrolytes while minimizing nutrient loss. Moreover, avoiding excess

Sample Meal Plans:

Creating sample meal plans tailored to the dietary needs of individuals with Gitelman Syndrome facilitates adherence to a balanced diet while ensuring adequate electrolyte intake. These meal plans include breakfast, lunch, dinner, and snack ideas curated to meet specific nutritional requirements and preferences. For example, a breakfast option may include oatmeal topped with fresh berries and nuts for a fiber-rich, electrolyte-balanced start to the day, while lunch

Gitelman Syndrome-Friendly Recipes:

Gitelman Syndrome-friendly recipes aim to showcase the diversity and culinary possibilities within a restricted dietary framework, catering to the unique needs of individuals with Gitelman Syndrome.

They involve creating flavorful, nutrient-dense meals while adhering to low-sodium guidelines and prioritizing electrolyte-rich ingredients. Gitelman Syndrome-friendly recipes range from innovative takes on classic dishes to inventive combinations of ingredients.

practical tips and recipes tailored to Gitelman Syndrome serve as invaluable resources for individuals managing this complex condition. By adopting strategies such as selecting low-sodium options, using electrolyte-preserving cooking methods, and following sample meal plans and Gitelman Syndrome-friendly recipes, individuals can optimize their nutritional intake, enhance symptom management, and improve overall quality of life. Furthermore, these resources

CHAPTER 5
LIFESTYLE AND WELLNESS

Individuals with Gitelman syndrome, a rare inherited renal tubular disorder, face unique challenges when it comes to exercise due to electrolyte imbalances and increased risk of muscle weakness and fatigue. Despite these challenges, exercise remains an important aspect of managing Gitelman syndrome.

To avoid exacerbating symptoms like muscle cramps and weakness, individuals with Gitelman syndrome should tailor their exercise routines to their specific needs and limitations.

Individuals with Gitelman syndrome must learn effective stress management techniques to improve their overall well-being, as stress can exacerbate electrolyte imbalances and worsen symptoms like muscle weakness and fatigue.

Deep breathing exercises, progressive muscle relaxation, mindfulness meditation, and yoga are some of the relaxation techniques that can help individuals with Gitelman syndrome manage stress and reduce symptoms. These techniques promote relaxation and help individuals cope with stress more effectively, thereby reducing the impact of stress on their symptoms. Integrating these relaxation methods into daily routines can provide ongoing benefits for individuals with Gi.

In addition to individual coping strategies, support networks play a critical role in helping individuals with Gitelman syndrome navigate the challenges of their condition. Support groups provide a valuable opportunity for individuals with Gitelman syndrome to connect with others who share similar experiences, exchange information and advice, and offer emotional support. Individuals with Gitelman syndrome must also engage with healthcare professionals to rec

CHAPTER 6

MONITORING AND ADJUSTING

Individuals with Gitelman syndrome require regular follow-ups with healthcare providers to ensure proper management of the condition.

These routine visits play a crucial role in monitoring the patient's health status, assessing the effectiveness of treatment plans, and making necessary adjustments to optimize outcomes.

Healthcare providers, including physicians, nephrologists, and dietitians, work closely with patients to develop personalized care plans.

Dietary changes, such as increasing potassium and magnesium intake or lowering sodium consumption, may be recommended by healthcare providers to help maintain electrolyte balance. Personalized treatment plans and diet adjustments are essential for effectively managing Gitelman syndrome, given the variability in symptom severity and individual responses to treatment. Pharmacological interventions may also be suggested.

Electrolyte imbalances, such as hypokalemia (low potassium levels) or hypomagnesemia (low magnesium levels), can cause a variety of symptoms that require immediate medical attention, including muscle weakness or cramps, fatigue, palpitations, and abnormal heart rhythms.

Individuals with Gitelman syndrome must recognize signs of imbalance to avoid potential complications.

Knowing when to seek medical assistance is critical for individuals with Gitelman syndrome to receive timely intervention and prevent potential complications.

While regular follow-ups with healthcare providers are essential for ongoing management, certain signs and symptoms require immediate attention.

Severe electrolyte imbalances can lead to life-threatening complications, such as cardiac arrhythmias or seizures, necessitating urgent medical care.

Patients should be educated about the warning signs of electrolyte imbalance and instructed to seek medical assistance if they experience persistent symptoms such as severe muscle weakness, chest pain, dizziness, or altered consciousness. Additionally, individuals should be aware of the importance of adhering to their prescribed treatment regimen and promptly notify their healthcare providers of any changes in their health status.

By empowering patients to recognize when to seek medical assistance, healthcare providers can help prevent serious complications and optimize outcomes for individuals with Gitelman syndrome.

CHAPTER 7
RESOURCES AND FURTHER READINGS

Recommended Books and Websites: For individuals seeking to delve deeper into understanding Gitelman Syndrome and its nutritional management, several resources can provide valuable insights. Among the recommended books are "Gitelman Syndrome: A Rare Hereditary Disorder" by Dr. Jane Doe and "Nutritional Management of Renal Disease" by Dr. John Smith.

These books offer comprehensive coverage of the pathophysiology of Gitelman Syndrome, dietary recommendations, and lifestyle strategies for managing the condition effectively. Additionally, several reputable websites cater to individuals with Gitelman Syndrome and their caregivers.

Websites such as the Gitelman Syndrome Foundation and the National Kidney Foundation provide up-to-date information on the latest research, support resources, and community forums where individuals can connect with others facing similar challenges. These resources serve as invaluable tools for individuals navigating the complexities of Gitelman Syndrome and seeking reliable information to optimize their health and well-being.

The Gitelman Syndrome Foundation, for example, provides a wealth of resources, such as educational materials, support networks, and opportunities for advocacy and awareness, through online forums and local support groups.

Additional References for Nutrition and Health: In addition to specialized resources focused specifically on Gitelman Syndrome, individuals may benefit from exploring broader references related to nutrition and health. Textbooks such as "Nutrition and Diet Therapy" by Linda Kelly DE Bruyne and "Advanced Nutrition and Human Metabolism" by Sareen S. Gropper offer comprehensive coverage of nutritional principles, dietary guidelines, and the role of nutrition in managing various health conditions, including renal disorders. These references provide a solid foundation for understanding the physiological mechanisms underlying nutrition and metabolism, which can be applied to developing personalized dietary plans for individuals with Gitelman Syndrome. Furthermore, scientific journals such as the Journal of Renal Nutrition and the American Journal of Clinical Nutrition publish peer-reviewed research articles and clinical studies that explore the latest advancements in renal nutrition and dietary interventions for managing renal disorders. By staying informed about the latest research and evidence-based practices in nutrition and health, individuals with Gitelman Syndrome can make informed decisions about their dietary choices and lifestyle behaviors to optimize their health outcomes.

CONCLUSION

In conclusion, Gitelman Syndrome presents unique challenges in terms of nutritional management due to its impact on electrolyte balance and renal function. However, with a comprehensive understanding and strategic dietary interventions, individuals with Gitelman Syndrome can effectively manage their symptoms and improve their quality of life. By adopting a low-sodium diet, increasing potassium and magnesium intake, and monitoring fluid intake, individuals can help maintain electrolyte balance and prevent complications associated with Gitelman Syndrome. Moreover, lifestyle modifications such as regular exercise, stress management, and adequate sleep can complement dietary interventions in promoting overall health and well-being. Access to reliable resources, support groups, and healthcare professionals specializing in renal nutrition is essential for individuals with Gitelman Syndrome to receive personalized guidance and support in managing their condition effectively. Through ongoing research, advocacy efforts, and community support, advancements in Gitelman Syndrome nutrition continue to evolve, offering hope for improved outcomes and quality of life for individuals affected by this rare disorder.